How to make

Salves

Book Two of the Herbal Preparations Series

By Starr Morgayne

How to make Salves by Starr Morgayne

How to make
Salves

Book Two of the Herbal Preparations Series

Written by Starr Morgayne

Cover Design by Starr Morgayne

Published by

Dark Moon Press

P.O. Box 11496

Fort Wayne, Indiana 46858-1496

www.DarkMoonPress.com

DarkMoon@DarkMoonPress.com

ISBN 10: 1495381072

ISBN-13: 978-1495381072

Health & Fitness/Herbal Medicine

How to make Salves by Starr Morgayne

How to make Salves by Starr Morgayne

Other Books by Starr Morgayne

Bewitching Beauty; Bringing out your inner Goddess, naturally

How to Make Infusions and Decoctions; Book One in the Herbal Preparations Series

How to Make Tinctures and Glycerites; Book Three in the Herbal Preparations Series

How to Make Lotions and Creams; Book Four in the Herbal Preparations Series

How to make Salves by Starr Morgayne

Disclaimer

The information contained within this book is presented solely for general informational purposes only. Nothing contained in this book is intended to constitute, nor should it be considered, medical advice. It should not serve as a substitute for the advice of a physician or other qualified health care provider. I make no assurances of the information being suited to your medical needs and, to the maximum extent allowed by law, disclaim any and all warranties and liabilities related to your use of any of the information and/or recipes obtained from within these pages. Please make sure to keep in mind any allergies and/or dietary concerns when working with plants and other ingredients.

The information provided in this book should not be considered complete, nor should it be relied on to suggest a course of treatment for a particular individual, nor is it intended to refer you to a particular medical professional or health care provider. It should not be used as a substitute for a visit to, consultation with or the advice of a physician or other qualified health care provider.

Information obtained from within this book is not exhaustive and does not cover all diseases, ailments or physical conditions or their treatment. Should you have any health care related questions, call or see your physician or other qualified health care provider promptly. You should never disregard medical advice or delay in seeking it because of something you have read in this book.

How to make Salves by Starr Morgayne

How to make Salves by Starr Morgayne

How to make Salves by Starr Morgayne

Table of Contents

Introduction

Taking care of people and helping them heal has always interested me. I think that might stem from my grandmother being a nurse and my mother wanting to follow in those footsteps. I, however, went in a slightly different direction.

I was always curious about different plant life. My mother had a large garden where she grew many vegetables and I enjoyed helping her in the garden and smelling the vegetables as they grew.

My mother is very much a plant lover and so we had many houseplants all around. Because of this, one of my science fair projects in Junior High was studying the growth of plants and how outside stimuli affected them. One of the things that I found out is that talking to and playing music for them helped them grow immensely and to this day when I water my little lovelies I tell them how proud of them I am and how beautiful they're looking.

I very much enjoyed picking things from the garden and making meals out of it. The produce that I would walk along the aisles grazing upon always tasted so much better than the everyday grocery store fare.

My love of making things, as well as my love of herbs and other plants, grew as I got older. In my late teens I became interested in my Native American heritage. I began going to powwows and creating Native American style jewelry. This got me even more interested in how my ancestors lived. I began studying what foods they ate and how they healed themselves through food and natural medicines. This got me started with making teas, bath bags, salves, etc.

Thanks to random chance I met up with a woman who would change my life. Through her teachings I learned so much more. I slept in a tipi on her property many times. I picked St. John's Wort in her meadow, helped build an arch for the gourds in her garden, scraped a deer hide to get it ready for tanning, fed chickens, watched the sun rise and the rabbits hop across the field as the deer grazed, suffered through many a sweat lodge ceremony and loved every minute of it.

Since that time I have continued on with my study of herbs, alternative medicine, naturopathy (healing through food) and Native cultures.

My days now are spent caring for my zoo of animals, my family and creating even more salves, lotions, potions, brews, teas and anything else I can think of.

I wanted to write this book so that I can share with you, the reader, my love of everything natural as well as the knowledge I have gained throughout my time here.

Many of the things that we need to sustain ourselves, keep ourselves healthy and make ourselves beautiful is right in our own backyards, sometimes literally.

This is, in my opinion, a healthier and more harmonious way of going about things. It is also more in accordance with our own bodies and helps them work in a more natural manner.

The information contained in this book has come from many different sources too numerous to name. In all of these years I have grown, researched and learned more than I could imagine. I hope that I can encourage you to do the same.

If you have any questions about ingredients or definitions of terms used within these pages I have included a glossary of terms as well as an ingredient list at the end of this book. Many of your questions may be answered there.

If you cannot find the answer to your questions within these pages, I encourage you to contact me through my publisher, Dark Moon Press (DarkMoon@DarkMoonPress.com), Facebook (https://www.facebook.com/StarrMorgayne), or research the information on your own.

How to Make Salves

Salves (also known as balms or ointments) are a mixture of infused oils and a thickener. When we think of balms and ointments we tend to think of something with a softer consistency. In order to make a balm or ointment just use less of the thickening agent when preparing your salve.

The thickening agents that I have used are hydrogenated vegetable oil (vegetable shortening), Coconut Oil and beeswax. Hydrogenated vegetable oil (vegetable shortening) and Coconut Oil are great to use if you are making a vegan product because vegans use no animal products; however, I prefer to use beeswax. It makes a nice smooth salve and has a thicker consistency than the hydrogenated vegetable oil (vegetable shortening) or even the Coconut Oil, most of the time. The downside of using Coconut Oil is that it will turn to liquid at 77° or above. I will get into more on using the thickeners later in this book.

Let's start with the first step: making the oil infusion.

Oil Infusions

If you have the first book in this series, *How To Make Infusions and Decoctions*, you will already have this information, however, they may be some different things mentioned in this book that are updated.

Infused oils should NOT be confused with essential oils. Essential oils are extremely concentrated and are sometimes combined with carrier oils like the ones used in our infusions.

True essential oils are strictly oils extracted from the plant material and contain no carrier oils. Many should not be used internally or applied directly to the skin. Many companies that you find in some craft stores will try to sell an "essential oil" that is actually fragrance oil (often an oil infused with an artificial fragrance) or essential oil diluted in carrier oil (creating an infused oil) to make it more affordable. Essential oils do not go rancid but should still be stored in a cool, dark place to maintain their potency. They can lose their therapeutic qualities over time. Carrier oils will go rancid and should also be stored in a cool, dark place.

When making oil infusions you can use lots of different oils. My favorite is Extra Virgin Olive Oil but you can use Olive Oil, Canola Oil, Sunflower Oil, Sesame Oil, Castor Oil, Almond Oil, Avocado Oil, Jojoba Oil or a plethora of other oils.

Different oils have all different properties when applied to the skin. Some, like Almond Oil, soak into the skin more readily than others and so shouldn't be used for massage oils or anything that requires the oil remain on top of the skin for a length of time. Other oils, like Olive Oil, are good for this purpose because they take a little longer to be absorbed.

These oils also have different shelf lives. Please check to see what the shelf life is of the particular oil that you're using so that you can store it properly. Extra Virgin Olive Oil, stored in an unopened container, can last three years (though the average shelf life is about 2 years, as seen in the list below). Keeping the oils away from light, heat and ail will help to extend their shelf lives.

Here is a list of different oils you might like to use and their average shelf life:

Almond Oil ~ 1 year
Avocado Oil ~ 1 year
Jojoba Oil ~ 2+ years
Olive Oil ~ 2 years
Sesame Oil ~ 1 year
Sunflower Oil ~ 1 year

You can combine different oils for their different properties also. Some of the oil with a longer shelf life can help to extend the shelf life of the ones that don't last quite as long.

Almond Oil, or Sweet Almond Oil, soaks into the skin pretty quickly and is better used for things that you don't need to stay on top of the skin for an extended length of time. It is a thin oil that has a slight nutty aroma. It is a good oil to use for lip balms (which are a form of salve).

Avocado Oil has lots of vitamins A, D and E. It also contains protein and amino acids. All of these are great for mature skin. It is a good nourishing oil for both skin and hair. It is a thick oil and can leave a waxy coat on the skin. It is usually mixed with another oil when used for skin care. Do not refrigerate.

Jojoba Oil is a good choice for people with acne prone skin. It is technically a wax but is very close in composition to our skin's natural oils. It is also said to have anti-inflammatory properties. It is good for all skin types and readily absorbed.

Olive Oil is very mild and moisturizing. I like to use Extra Virgin Olive Oil for a lot of what I do. It's affordable and works well for lotions, creams and massage oils. The downside of using Olive Oil is that it does have a fragrance to it which can overpower other scents. It can also cause an allergic reaction in some people.

Sesame Oil, also known as sesame seed oil, is a thick oil with a slight aroma and can have a dark color. It is best blended with other oils and very good for massage. It is also said to have anti-inflammatory properties and is good for all skin types.

Sunflower Oil is a good, all-purpose oil. Try to get unrefined if possible. It is a thin oil with a faint, sweet scent. It can be almost odorless. It is great for those who are allergic to nuts or who may have delicate skin. It is rich in vitamins and minerals.

If any of your carrier oils develop a strong bitter aroma they have gone rancid and should be disposed of. The shelf lives will vary quite a bit based on how an oil was processed and how it has been stored.

As with anything that you are going to put on or in your body, you want to make sure that there are no allergies or dietary concerns with the oils that you use.

To protect your infusions when they are finished you are going to want to keep them away from heat and light. There are many places where you can get amber or cobalt blue colored bottles to store your infusions in.

Always make sure to do your research when making any sort of herbal preparation. Make sure that the herb(s) you are using are not poisonous or that whomever may be using the preparation doesn't have any allergies to the herbs that you have used.

Using Fresh Plants

If you are using fresh plants, make sure you know exactly what plant you are using and what that plant does as well as what parts of the plant are best to use for what you are trying to accomplish. If you use the wrong plant because it looks like another, or you're not sure what it is, the effects can be harmful and even, sometimes, fatal. If you're using the wrong part of the plant, even if you are using the correct plant, you may not get the results that you you're looking for in the preparation that you are creating. You may need the bark instead of the leaves or you might need the root

Collecting Lemon Balm from my yard to make an infusion.

instead of the petals of the flower. Always make sure you've done your homework before putting anything together.

Because fresh plant material still has moisture in it there is a possibility that with certain recipes (such as infused oils) you may get some mold growth. In order to avoid this make sure to cover all of the plant material with oil and you can also add a natural preservative such as Vitamin E or Grapefruit Seed Extract while you are storing your infusion.

Using Dried Plants

If you are using dried plant material you want to make sure that it has maintained its color and scent. Crush or rub a little in your hands and smell it to make sure if

 you need to. If you aren't able to crush and smell the herbs take a look at their color. If the herbs are dull and brown looking they have lost their potency. If the herb is meant to be brown, such as cinnamon or cloves, look at the intensity of the color. Herbs that maintain a bright color will usually have maintained their potency as well. Another thing to remember when using dried herbs is that you'll usually want to replace them every 6 months or so. I have been able to keep herbs for longer than that but you always need to check the color and scent. Often times I'll use older herbs for crafts where the potency is not such a big issue.

If you're using a recipe that calls for a certain amount of fresh herbs you'll need less of the dried herbs. The ratio most commonly used is 2 to 1 (or ½ the amount of dried herb as compared to fresh). If your recipe calls for two tablespoons of fresh herb then you should be able to use one tablespoon of dried herb and vice versa.

Some plants work just as well in dried form as they do fresh but some do not. In some cases you will need the vital oils from the fresh plant in order to accomplish the goal of whatever you are creating.

Always make sure to store your herbs away from light and heat in order to keep them fresher longer. Storing them in a cabinet can help with this. My family often jokes that I need my own "herb cabinet" the size of a small bedroom.

Powdered herbs will lose their efficacy the quickest. Once the herbs are ground into a powder their essential oils will dissipate rapidly. I don't usually use powdered herbs to make infusions. If I do need to use the powdered form of an herb I will usually either dry it myself or purchase it in dried form then grind it into a powder with my coffee grinder.

Some herbs have properties that are better extracted in water and some properties that are better extracted through oil. Common Plantain is one example. You can use a water infusion and an oil infusion, separately of course, to extract both types of properties from the plant and then combine them, along with an emulsifying agent, into a healing cream.

At the end of this book you will find recipes in which to use your oil infusions to make salves. I hope you enjoy them and that it inspires you to come up with some recipes of your own.

Solar Oil Infusions

To make a solar infusion (also known as a cold infusion because direct heat is not applied) with oil you will want to use the same process as you would if you were making a solar water infusion.

A solar infusion uses the heat of the sun to warm the oils so that they will extract what is needed out of the plants. To do this you take a clean, sterile jar, fill it with plant material, cover the plant material in the oil of your choice, get as much air bubbles out as you can (you can use a chopstick or something similar to poke around the outside of the plant material to release the air pockets), seal the jar with a clean, sterile lid and sit it on a sunny, warm windowsill for 2-4 weeks depending on the weather. Put a label on the jar with all of the information you will need: the name of the herb you are using, the type of infusion (water, oil, etc.), the date which you started the infusion and the date which the infusion should be ready to use.

Make sure that when you pour the oil you are using over the herbs that you fill it until the oil reaches just over the top of the herbs. All of the plant material must be covered to help avoid any growth of bacteria or fungi. Every day you will want to turn or shake your bottle at least once and make sure that the plant material is still covered by the oil. If you use dry herbs the plant material may swell as it becomes rehydrated.

After the appropriate amount of time, you will want to remove the jar from its sunny location and strain the plant material from the liquid using cheesecloth, a coffee filter, a French Press, or any other way you feel comfortable. If you're using cheesecloth or something similar you can wrap it up like a little bundle, twist it up the top so nothing comes out and squeeze it with your hands to get as much of the oil out as possible. It is a messy process but well worth it. You want to make sure that you have been able to remove any of the particles left over from the plant material itself. You can then compost your leftover plant material and store your infusion or use it.

If you would like to make a stronger concentration of oil, you can put more herbs in the jar and pour the already infused oil back over them to repeat the steeping process. You can continue to do this repeatedly until the oil is as concentrated as you would like.

If you want to add a natural preservative to your infused oils you can use some Vitamin E oil, Grapefruit Seed Extract or even Tincture of Benzoin. You should only need a very small amount of any of these preservatives depending on the amount of infusion you are adding the preservative to. There are other natural oils that you can use as a preservative too. I make a particular foot lotion that I add both Vitamin E oil and Tea Tree Essential Oil to because both act as preservatives and are beneficial for the type of lotion I am making.

The Stove or Fire Method

If you want to infuse your oils on a stove or over a fire you will want to place your plant material into a pot and cover it with oil. Place the pot over the fire (or on the burner). Be very careful with this method because you could end up cooking the herbs. You don't want to cook them; you just want to infuse the oil with the essences of the herbs. Place the pot on the lowest heat setting possible. You want to heat the oil enough to infuse the herbs but you don't want to fry them. Let the herbs infuse for about 3 hours but keep an eye on them to make sure the heat is not too high. When they are thoroughly infused remove them from the heat and allow the infusion to cool off. Once it's cool you can strain out the plant material. At this time you can add in the Vitamin E oil or

Grapefruit Seed Extract.

Another stove or fire method is done by using a double boiler or bain-marie. There is less chance of frying your plant material if you use this method. You can either buy a double boiler or make one yourself.

Merriam-Webster defines a bain-marie as "a cooking utensil containing heated water in which food in smaller pots is cooked — compare double boiler". To make a double boiler you will need a glass or ceramic bowl that will fit in a pot. I like to use a glass bowl that's edges sit on the edge of the large pot. You will then fill the large pot about halfway with water and place the glass bowl in the pot. It should rest on top of the water. Place the plant material inside the bowl and then pour the oil over it. Turn on the heat as you did in the first method and allow it to steep for the same amount of time. The water acts as a barrier to keep the plant material from frying in the oil, using indirect heat, but it still needs to be watched carefully.

Again, remove the infusion from the heat and allow it to cool before straining it. You can then add your preservative.

The Slow Cooker Method

Pouring oil over herbs.

The slow cooker method is my preferred method of infusing oils. It is a great method for those who may be doing many things at once (which I find is often the case with myself). It is still possible to fry your plant material using this method though it is less likely.

I use a small two quart slow cooker for this particular method. It has a "warm" setting and

Lemon Balm after infusing in oil in the slow cooker.

makes the oil in good sized batches. It is basically the same process. You place your plant material in the bottom of the slow cooker and cover it with the oil. If your slow cooker has a "warm" setting you will want to use that. If your slow cooker doesn't have a "warm" setting you will want to place it on the lowest setting possible. I have seen a very small accessory for the slow cooker called a "Little Dipper" that could possibly be used for this purpose also, though I have not tried it myself.

You can leave your plant material in the slow cooker for a few hours (usually around two to four) but make sure to check on it periodically.

When the oil is ready, turn off your slow cooker and allow the infusion to cool before you try straining it. If you don't let it cool you could burn yourself and hot oil burns are nasty ones.

You can make your oils stronger and more concentrated by using the same method as with the solar oil infusions. Just strain the oil from the plant material and add more plant material to the already infused oil, then repeat whatever process you used to infuse the oil the first time.

In the picture to the left you can see where I have placed the oil infusion in the French Press. You can also use a mesh strainer, cheesecloth, a coffee filter, or other similar ways to strain your oils.

In the picture on the right I am starting to press the filter down so that it strains the plant material from the oil.

In this picture (left) you can see that the filter is all the way to the bottom of the press and the clear, strained liquid is above the filter.

In the next photo you can see the strained, infused oil being poured into a glass jar for storage. I have used a clear glass jar for this picture to make it easier to see, however, you would want to use an amber or other dark colored jar to store your herbal infused oils in so that they remain safe from light.

Oil infusions can be used in foods (as a marinade or salad dressing depending on what herbs you've used and if they are safe to ingest), made into lotions, creams, salves, cleaning products and massage and/or body oils. There are a plethora of uses for infused oils. Make sure to store them in a cool, dark place. Using a brown, cobalt blue, or other dark colored storage bottle or jar can extend their shelf life. Another thing that can extend their shelf life is using natural preservatives.

For many of my salves, lotions and creams I use a combination of Calendula Petals and Comfrey (leaf and/or root) in my infused oils. My reason for doing so is because Comfrey helps to regenerate cells and Calendula Petals are anti-inflammatory, antiseptic, antifungal, antibacterial, cleansing, softening, smoothing as well as regenerative. Calendula also accelerates healing.

Adding the thickener

Once the oil has cooled and you have strained out all of the bits of plant material, and made sure you have the concentration of oil that you would like, you can begin adding the thickening agent.

As I said before, my favorite thickening agent is beeswax but hydrogenated vegetable oil (vegetable shortening) or Coconut Oil can be used also. If you like, you can even use lard or tallow.

Hydrogenated vegetable oil (vegetable shortening), Coconut Oil, lard and tallow all come in forms that are fairly easy to use as is. Coconut Oil is usually solid at room temperature but turns to liquid at around 77°F.

Cocoa Butter and Shea butter can add some great healing and skin softening qualities to a salve but aren't normally used in large enough quantities to make a thick salve.

Beeswax comes in a couple of different forms. If you buy beeswax in a cake (as shown in the picture on the left) you will want to grate it into small slivers so that it will melt easier.

If you are using lard or tallow you may have to cut it into smaller chunks for the same reason.

Most often I buy my beeswax in bead form (shown in the picture on the right) because it saves me time since I don't have to grate it to make it ready to use.

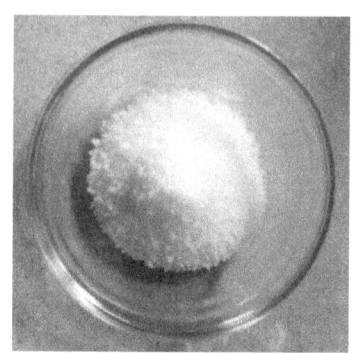

Your next step would then be to put the oil back on a very slight heat, just enough to warm it up, and slowly add in the beeswax or other thickening agent. Keep it

on the heat until the thickener is completely melted. The picture on the left shows the beeswax poured into the melted oil. I then put the glass bowl on a pot of water to create a bain-marie (double boiler) and melt the beeswax.

Once everything is liquefied, and you have made sure it is slightly cooled, you can add in whichever preservative you have chosen to use; Vitamin E Oil, Grapefruit Seed Extract, etc. You can also add in any essential oils, honey, or other additives that you don't want to add in before the heating process because they might be affected negatively by the heat.

Once you have everything you want incorporated into the oil you can pour it into your containers.

The picture below shows the, still liquid, salve poured

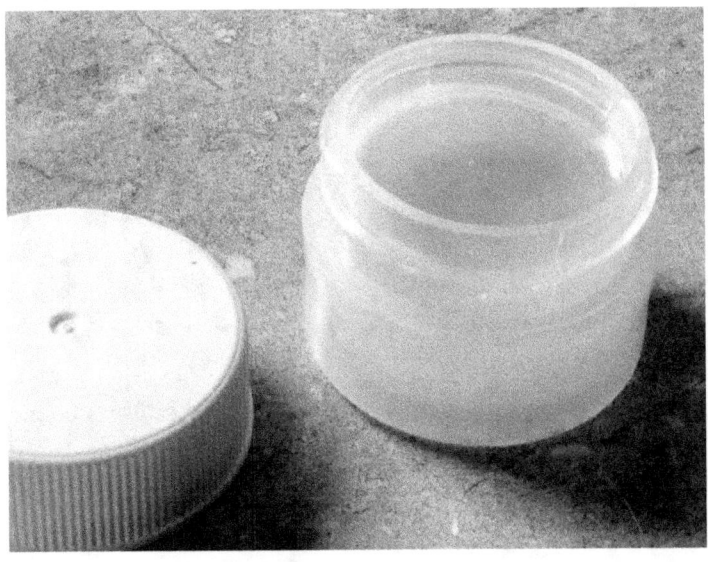

into the container. At this point you want to leave the lid off of the container and allow the salve to cool. Once it cools you will see if you need to add any more liquid salve to the container because there can be some shrinkage.

The picture on the next page shows the salve after it has cooled. As you can see there is a slight dip in the center of the salve but not enough to need to add any more to it. It is now ready to place the lid on and label it.

When it comes to using beeswax or other thickeners, there are several different ideas on how much to use. I have heard an 8:1 oil to beeswax ratio is a good one. I have also heard 2:1 or even 3:1. I have (what some consider to be) a bad habit of not measuring things out so I just put some beeswax in, heat it gently until the beeswax is completely melted into the oil and let it sit. If it's still too runny after it cools I reheat it gently again and add a little more beeswax. If it's too hard I'll, again, reheat it gently and add a little more of the leftover oil. Keeping a bit of your infused oil out is always helpful in case you get a little carried away with the thickening agent. You may have to experiment with this a couple of times to get it precise. It really depends on how hard you want your end product to be. Based on what you want to use the salve for, you may want a harder salve or a softer salve. You really just have to use your best judgment to determine what you want it to end up like.

When making your salves you can use just essential oils or a combination of herb infused oils and essential oils. The salves that I personally make are usually a combination of the two.

When using just essential oils (or a combination of herb infused oil and essential oils), as stated earlier, you will want to combine your oil and thickening agent and when it cools slightly (but before it solidifies) add in your essential oils and mix them well. If you put additives like essential oils or honey into your salve before it cools enough the heat can destroy some of the beneficial elements that the additives contain.

There are many different uses for this method of making herbal preparations. You can even use it for things that we don't think of as salves, such as deodorant sticks, lip balms or solid perfumes. There are tons of uses for this type of preparation so use your imagination and get creative.

Recipes

Basic Healing Salve

This is a basic salve recipe that can be used for any type of salve that you would like to make. You can use several different combinations.

Herb infused oil (I use Calendula Petals and Comfrey)
Enough beeswax or other thickening agent to solidify

Infuse your herbs into the oil following the steps previously shown in this book. Melt the thickening agent separately. Combine the oil and the melted thickening agent together and mix well. Allow to solidify.

You can add many different ingredients to the infused oil (such as Lavender, Peppermint, Tea Tree) to make salves for different uses. You can even use the basic salve recipe and add ingredients such as Peppermint Essential Oil, Vanilla Extract, Cocoa Butter (this would be a partial thickening agent also) or melted chocolate or honey and turn this salve into a delightful lip balm.

Healing Herbal Baby Balm

All three of the herbs used in this salve have been shown to be powerful yet gentle. Because of this, the salve can be used to help with diaper rash or act as a moisturizer for very dry skin. It can even help with small cuts and scratches.

2 cups Extra Virgin Olive Oil (or Almond Oil)

1/3 cup Comfrey

1/3 cup Chamomile

1/3 cup Lavender

6 capsules Vitamin E (or ½ tablespoon Vitamin E oil)

Enough beeswax to make salve the right consistency

Combine the herbs and oil using any of the methods listed previously in this book. After you have the herbs infused into the oil, have made sure it is cooled and strained you can then add in the Vitamin E oil. Now, you'll want to put the oil back on a very slight heat, just enough to warm it up and slowly add in the beeswax until it is completely melted. You can then pour the salve into your prepared containers and let it sit to solidify.

Baby Bottom Balm

This balm has herbs in it that will soften and soothe baby's skin.

2 cups Extra Virgin Olive Oil (or Almond Oil)

1/3 cup Calendula

1/3 cup Rose Petals

1/3 cup Chamomile

6 capsules Vitamin E (or ½ tablespoon Vitamin E oil)

A few drops Lavender essential Oil

Enough beeswax to make salve the right consistency

This is made pretty much exactly like the previous baby balm. Combine the herbs and oil using any of the methods listed previously in this book. After you have the herbs infused into the oil, have made sure it is cooled and strained you can then add in the Vitamin E oil. Now, you'll want to put the oil back on a very slight heat, just enough to warm it up and slowly add in the beeswax until it is completely melted. You can then pour the salve into your prepared containers and let it sit to solidify.

Gently apply to baby's bottom after a bath.

Sore Muscle Salve

10 drops Peppermint essential oil

10 drops Eucalyptus essential oil

5 drops Clove essential oil

¼ Cup Extra Virgin Olive Oil

About 1 tablespoon of beeswax

Heat the Olive Oil and beeswax in a double boiler over low heat. Stir the mixture until the wax is completely melted. Remove from the heat and let it cool slightly. Stir in the essential oils, and pour the mixture into small glass or metal containers to solidify.

To use this salve just scoop a little out of the container and rub it onto the area where the muscle is sore. Massage it in deeply so that the oils can work their magic. The Clove will help to numb the area and relieve some of the pain while the Peppermint and Eucalyptus add a little heat and cooling at the same time.

This salve can also be used as a decongestant when rubbed on the chest and/or under the nose.

Triple Antibiotic Ointment

10 drops Tea Tree essential oil

10 drops Lavender essential oil

5 drops Lemon essential oil

5 drops or 1/8 tsp Vitamin E oil or raw, organic honey

¼ cup Extra Virgin Olive Oil

About 1 tablespoon of beeswax

Heat the Olive Oil and beeswax in a double boiler over low heat. Stir until wax is melted. Remove from heat. Let cool slightly. Stir in essential oils and Vitamin E Oil or Honey, and pour into small glass or metal containers to solidify.

Tea Tree essential oil is antimicrobial, antiseptic, antiviral, antibacterial and antifungal. Lavender essential oil is analgesic, antiseptic, anti-inflammatory, and antibacterial. Lemon essential oil is antifungal, antibacterial, antiviral, astringent, anti-inflammatory, and immune stimulant. Because of all the properties of each of these oils this salve is a wonderful wound healer over all.

Cold Sore Lip Balm

Lemon Balm leaves, dried

¼ cup Almond Oil

1/8 tsp raw, organic honey

10 drops Tea Tree essential oil

5 drops Camphor essential oil

About 1 tablespoon of beeswax

Infuse the Almond Oil with the Lemon Balm leaves. Strain the infused oil and add to a double boiler with the beeswax. Heat enough to melt the beeswax and remove from heat. Let cool slightly. Add in the honey and essential oils. Pour into lip balm containers.

Lemon Balm and Tea Tree are antiviral. The Camphor in this recipe acts as an anesthetic and will help to numb the area. Honey has many healing properties and is a good additive for this lip balm.

Solid Perfume

Herb(s) of choice (optional)

Almond Oil

essential oil or fragrance oil of choice

thickening agent of choice

Infuse the Almond Oil with the herbs of your choice if you decide you would like to use herbs. Strain the infused oil and add to a double boiler with the thickening agent. Heat enough to melt the melt the thickening agent and remove from heat. Let cool slightly. Add in the essential oils or fragrance oils. Pour into containers. Any small container will do for this really. You can use lip balm containers. I have even heard of people using old contact lens cases as lip balm, solid perfume or salve containers.

I didn't add any measurements to this recipe because you should be able to decide for yourself how thick and how concentrated you would like your solid perfume to be.

Afterword

Many people today are not only concerned about the environment but also about their own health and more conscious about what they are putting in and on their bodies.

We have come to be a society that tends to rely on synthetic chemicals. Many of these synthetic chemicals originate from natural sources. Unfortunately, these natural sources have been taken apart, studied and the components with the desired effect have been isolated. The reason that this is a bad thing is because that the plants these components come from contain other components that work in harmony with each other. When you have a drug that causes side effects the natural source that the drug was taken from probably has other things in it to counteract those side effects. Instead of using those natural sources to harmoniously heal ourselves we end up taking pill after pill to combat a disease or illness and then to combat the side effects that the first pill caused.

Because of the recent trend toward healing the earth and using more natural products, many companies have put out products that use buzz words like "organic" and "natural". The sad thing is that your basic consumer will probably assume that because these words are listed on the label it means that this is a good for the environment product or something that doesn't have harmful additives or chemicals. Sadly, this is not the case. If you look closely at the label you may find that the product you're looking at with "organic" on the label only has one ingredient in it that is actually organic. The rest of the ingredients may be the same as every other similar product on the shelf. The same goes for those products labeled "natural".

In my life I use a combination of Naturopathy (healing through food), herbalism (healing through herbs) and aromatherapy (healing through scent). I am not against using allopathic medicine (what we have come to know as "traditional" medicine) for severe issues and/or emergencies. In those areas, allopathic medicine excels. I am a firm believer in integrated medicine. Integrated medicine is using a combination of natural healing modalities as well as allopathic medicine.

I hope that through my writing I can inspire you to take your health more personally and discover the things that you can do to create a better self in a more natural and harmonious manner.

Glossary of Terms

Analgesic – An analgesic is something that reduces pain

Anemia – Anemia is a condition in which your blood has a lower than normal number of red blood cells often referred to as an iron deficiency.

Anti-inflammatory – An anti-inflammatory is something that decreases inflammation.

Antibacterial – An antibacterial is something that destroys or inhibits the growth of bacteria.

Antimicrobial – An antimicrobial destroys or inhibits the growth of micro-organisms

Antioxidant – An antioxidant is a substance that reduces the damage that oxygen does to the tissue, usually caused by free radicals which are chemicals that attack the molecules in your skin.

Antiseptic – An antiseptic helps to prevent infection and to get rid of disease causing organisms.

Antispasmodic – An antispasmodic is used to help control the spasms of an involuntary muscle.

Antitussive – An antitussive is something that prevents or relieves a cough.

Antiviral – Something that is antiviral kills or prevents a virus from multiplying.

Astringent – An astringent is something that tightens soft tissue in order to slow the flow of secretions.

Carminative – A carminative is something that relieves flatulence (gas).

Decoction – A decoction is a type of infusion made by boiling roots, barks, seeds, stems, berries or heartier parts of plants

Demulcent – A demulcent is something soothing. Demulcents are usually used to soothe and soften inflamed skin.

Diaphoretic – A diaphoretic is something that has the power to increase perspiration (sweating).

Diuretic – A diuretic is something that has the power to increase urination.

Emmenagogue – An emmenagogue is something that stimulates or increases menstrual flow.

Emollient – An emollient is something that softens and moisturizes the skin. It is usually found in the form of a lotion or thick liquid.

Emulsifier – An emulsifier is something that allows ingredients that do not normally mix well to blend together. Example: oil and water.

Emulsion – An emulsion is a mixture of two (usually) liquids that don't normally mix. Example: oil and water.

Exfoliant – An exfoliant is an abrasive used to scrub the skin in order to remove dead skin cells and increase circulation.

Expectorant – Merriam-Webster defines an expectorant as "an agent that promotes the discharge or expulsion of mucus from the respiratory tract; *broadly* : an antitussive agent"

Extract – When we use the word "extract" we can either be referring to the process of creating something or the product itself. Merriam-Webster defines this process as "to withdraw (as a juice or fraction) by physical or chemical process" or "to treat with a solvent so as to remove a soluble substance". The finished product is sometimes referred to as "an extract".

Fungicide – A fungicide, simply put, is something that kills fungi.

Germicide – A germicide is something that kills germs.

Glycerite – A glycerite is an infusion or tincture made using the syrupy liquid glycerine as the base. Using glycerine instead of alcohol provide an alcohol-free alternative for children and those who may have issues with alcohol.

Humectant – A humectant holds water or moisture (in this case it is something that will hold moisture to the skin)

Inflammation – The symptoms of inflammation are usually pain, swelling, redness and heat.

Infusion – In the case of this book an infusion is what you get when you use a liquid to pull the needed constituents of an herb out of the plant matter and into the liquid. Example: tea

Maceration – Technically, maceration is the preparation of an extract by soaking the containing material in an organic solvent. This would include infusions, decoctions, tinctures etc. but in herbal terms it has come to mean, a cold infusion of herbs in water, oil or vinegar.

Nervine – The word nervine refers to something that is used to calm the nerves. A couple of examples would be Lavender and Valerian.

Poultice – A poultice is usually a warm, wet mass that is applied externally. It is most often on or in between cloth and used for inflamed areas of the body.

Salve – Merriam-Webster's Online Dictionary defines a salve as "an unctuous adhesive substance for application to wounds or sores." My definition of a salve is a mixture of herb infused oil with either beeswax, hydrogenated vegetable oil (like Crisco), Coconut Oil, or a similar substance.

Sebaceous Gland – The sebaceous glands are small glands in the skin which secrete a lubricating oily matter (sebum) into the hair follicles to lubricate the skin and hair.

Sebum – The natural oil secreted onto our skin by our sebaceous glands is known as sebum.

Steeping – Steeping is the process used to make an infusion. You would cover your plant matter with hot liquid and let it steep by letting it sit for however long is needed.

Tincture – A tincture is what you get when you infuse alcohol with plant matter.

Tools

Here is some information on some of the tools that you might like to have when you are making your own infusions and decoctions. You will want to make sure that you have separate items for making your medicinal preparations than you use for cooking because some of the ingredients you use may become absorbed by the tools and won't bode well for your cooking. If you are using essential oils remember that they can melt plastic.

Coffee Grinder ~ One of my favorite and most used tools is my coffee grinder. It is wonderful to use when I need to turn a dried herb into a powder.

Wooden Spoons ~ Wooden spoons are good for stirring your mixtures as they won't impart some of the impurities that using metal or plastic will. However, they can soak up smells and other components of what you are stirring them with.

Bowls ~ You'll need bowls to mix your ingredients. For some things you can use plastic bowls but for others you may want to use glass or ceramic.

Blender ~ A blender is good to have for making emulsions for lotions or creams. I have one blender for edible items and another for making my skin care products.

Cheesecloth ~ You can use this to make bath bags or tea bags. Cheesecloth can also be used for straining oils or other liquids through.

Coffee filters ~ Used for straining, similar to cheesecloth.

Double Boiler ~ In essence, this is two pans (or a pot and a glass bowl) put together. The one on the bottom has water in it. It is used to keep sensitive ingredients from getting too hot and burning. It is also known as a bain-marie.

Strainers ~ You can place cheesecloth or coffee filters within the strainer to strain the herb bits out of your infusions.

Measuring cups and spoons ~ You will need liquid measuring cups as well as those meant for solids.

Funnels ~ Funnels make filling bottles so much easier and a lot less messy. You will want to have several different sizes.

Mortar & Pestle ~ Every kitchen should have a mortar and pestle. It is good to use to grind up those things that you just can't get ground properly in a food processor or coffee grinder.

Pans ~ You can go with ceramic pans but you don't necessarily have to. Just remember that some metals may react adversely to some of the ingredients.

Bath Tea Bags ~ You don't necessarily have to have these but I love them. They're essentially large tea bags with drawstring closures. You can even use them to scrub yourself with or just hang them from your faucet for the water to flow through into the bath (after you've closed them and tied a knot in the drawstring at the opening of the bag and the end of the string). They're easily found at your local superstore or craft store. You can also sometimes substitute cheesecloth or even a wash cloth that is tied up around whatever you are using.

French Press ~ This is a somewhat fancy and completely optional item to have on hand. I like to use mine for straining oils and teas because I can squeeze out more of the infusion than I could with cheesecloth. The cheesecloth tends to soak up some of the infusion and can let small particles through.

Ingredients

Almond Oil, Sweet ~ Sweet Almond Oil (sometimes just called Almond Oil) is absorbed readily into the skin and makes a wonderful massage and carrier oil that is good for all skin types. It conditions, heals, revitalizes, smoothes and softens skin as well as being an emollient. One drawback is that it has a short shelf life.

Aloe Vera ~ Many of you are familiar with the Aloe Vera plant and its burn healing properties and its ability to help repair damaged tissue. Aloe Vera draws and holds oxygen to the skin which aids in the healing process. The gel from the leaf can be used but you can also find Aloe Vera juice in your local grocery store. It is soothing, softening, astringent and rejuvenating. It helps to draw out infections and heals skin irritations. It can also help to combat wrinkles. I like to use Aloe Vera juice instead of water when I make my lotions to give them an extra boost.

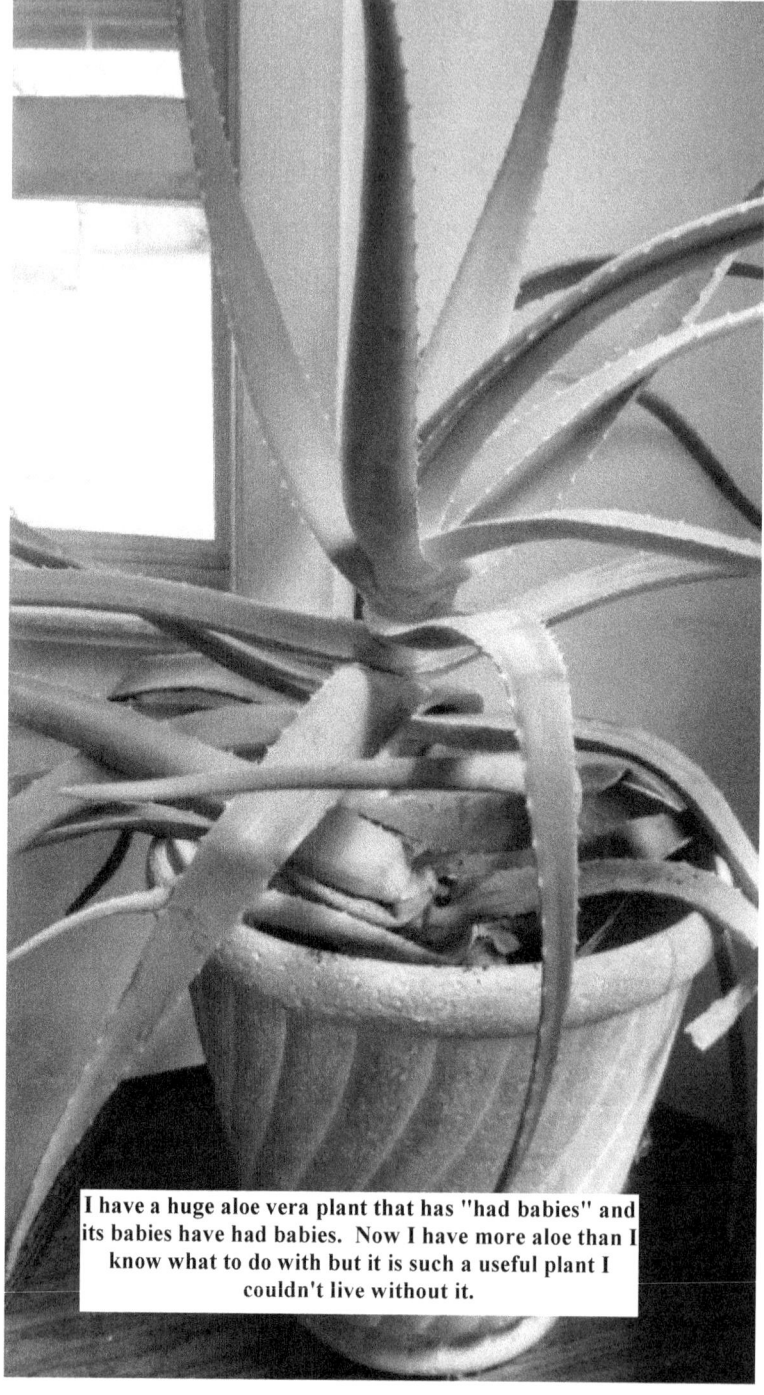

I have a huge aloe vera plant that has "had babies" and its babies have had babies. Now I have more aloe than I know what to do with but it is such a useful plant I couldn't live without it.

Apple Cider Vinegar ~ Apple Cider Vinegar is soothing and antiseptic. This valuable product helps to restore your skin's natural pH balance, relieve itchiness and is slightly astringent for those with normal to oily skin. It has been used for many years to help those afflicted with sunburn. Acetic acid is one of the main ingredients in Apple Cider Vinegar and has shown significant results for weight loss when used every day. It helps to create a more alkaline PH level within the system. It breaks up mucus within the body and cleanses the lymph nodes. It also helps relieve Candida because of the natural enzymes it contains.

Avocado ~ Avocado has nourishing and conditioning properties for both the skin and hair. The oil is used as an emollient. It is rich in proteins, minerals and vitamins and readily penetrates the skin. It is excellent for cracked or mature skin and heals, revitalizes and regenerates cells. Avocado Oil is excellent for face and massage oils. Avocadoes contain more Potassium than a banana and are also full of Vitamin D. The oils in the Avocado have been shown to reduce pain caused by Osteoarthritis. They have also been show to decrease "bad" cholesterol and increase "good" cholesterol.

Black Walnut ~ Black Walnut, specifically the hull, is often used for its antifungal properties as well as its astringency. It contains a high concentration of tannins which can also reduce pain and swelling. It is also

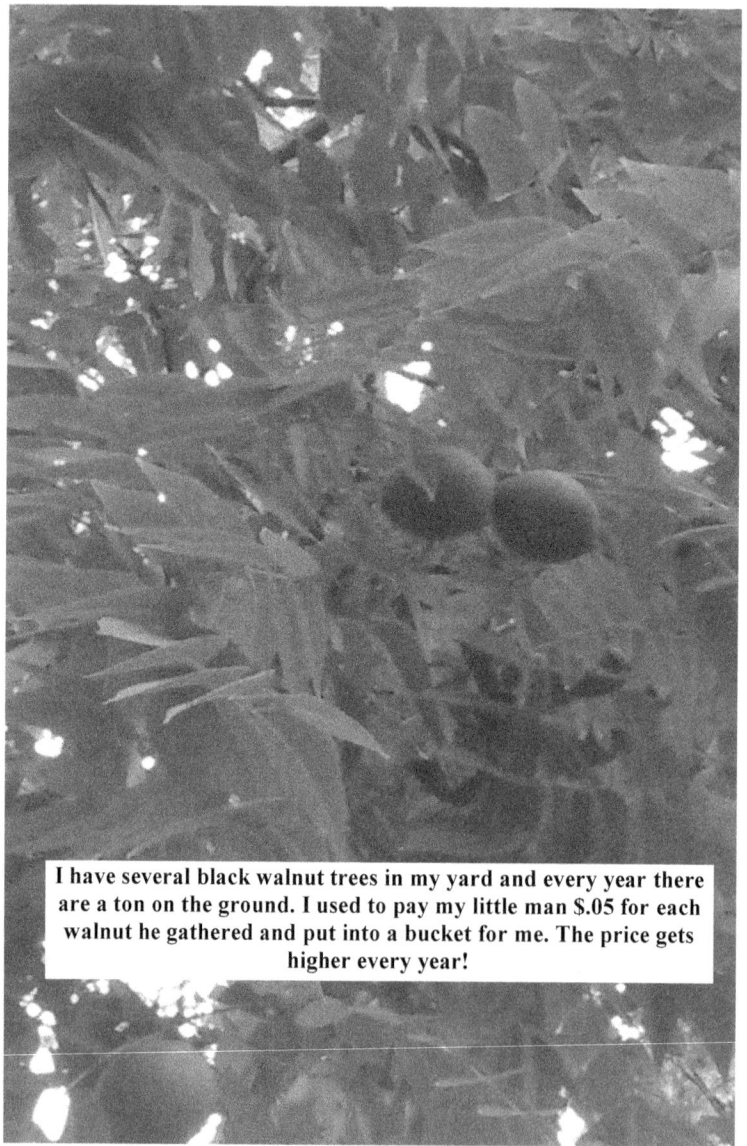

I have several black walnut trees in my yard and every year there are a ton on the ground. I used to pay my little man $.05 for each walnut he gathered and put into a bucket for me. The price gets higher every year!

antioxidant and antimicrobial. It is a natural laxative and a blood cleanser. If you've ever worked with Black Walnut Hull you are probably familiar with the fact that it can stain just about anything and has been used as a dye for centuries.

Burdock ~ Burdock is a plentiful (at least in my back yard) plant that has many different uses. You can use the leaves, roots and sometimes even the seeds. The roots are very bitter and can aid digestion, cleanse the liver, help absorb nutrients and eliminate waste. It can even help the liver's ability to metabolize hormones and therefore be used to treat hormonal imbalances such as estrogen dominance, endometriosis and Polycystic Ovarian Syndrome (PCOS). The root is sometimes sautéed with other vegetables in Oriental food dishes.

Calendula ~ Calendula (Calendula officinalis) is also known as Pot Marigold. It is very useful as a natural beauty tonic. It is anti-inflammatory, antiseptic, antifungal, antibacterial, cleansing, softening, smoothing as well as regenerative. It accelerates healing and can be used as a colorant. It is one of my favorite plants to use when making my own skin care products because it helps to tone and refresh the skin. It is useful in helping to prevent wrinkles and healing acne.

Here are the leaves of some Burdock plants in my yard. During their second year they will have long stalks with burrs at the end. This is how they got the name "Burdock".

Catnip ~ Catnip can be used in tea form to soothe and relax. It is even mild enough to give to small children. It is part of the Mint family and, as such, is said to help with digestive upsets in adults and to help with colic in children.

Chamomile, German ~ Chamomile tea is a great anti-inflammatory for pimples/zits/acne and is good for helping you relax and sleep. It is mildly astringent, diaphoretic, restorative and healing. Chamomile can also be used as a general anti-inflammatory and an antispasmodic.

Cinnamon ~ Cinnamon is antiseptic, astringent and stimulating. The powder can be used as an exfoliant but be careful because it can also be very irritating. Cinnamon has also been shown to lower the blood Sugar so it may be good for Diabetics. A popular way to take Cinnamon (other than on applesauce, oatmeal, or in a dessert) is to mix it with Honey and to eat a tablespoon of this infused syrup once a day. A study performed in Copenhagen found that this syrup helped with arthritis pains.

Clove ~ Cloves are antiseptic and their smell, usually brought out by using the essential oil, is used to calm and relieve stress. The oil is wonderful for toothaches as well. Whole Cloves (pictured below) are actually a flower bud.

Clover, Red ~ Red Clover is astringent (due to tannins) and anti-inflammatory. It is often used in combinations created for women's health issues. It is said that a tea made from Red Clover is good for symptoms of menopause.

Clover, White ~ White Clover is very common in my area. It is a cousin to the Red Clover. The young flowers are very sweet and can be eaten raw. It was used medicinally by Native Americans to heal and cleanse boils and wounds as well as made into to tea for coughs, colds and fevers.

Comfrey ~ Comfrey is used to soothe and lubricate dry skin. It is also helpful in cell regeneration. The leaf can be used as a compress for swelling and bruising. I use it, infused in oil with Calendula petals, as a base for many of my healing lotions, creams and salves.

Dandelion ~ Dandelions are often thought of as a common "weed" but, then again, so are many other useful plants. It can be used for food as well as medicine. It has been touted as a heartburn remedy, a coffee substitute (by roasting the roots) and as a cure-all for just about everything. Dandelion leaves are rich in minerals and have been said to aid in fighting off Osteoporosis. It is said that drinking a tea made of the Dandelion leaves can increase mobility and reduce stiffness. It is also thought to be most helpful for the liver for which it is a detoxifier and a strengthener.

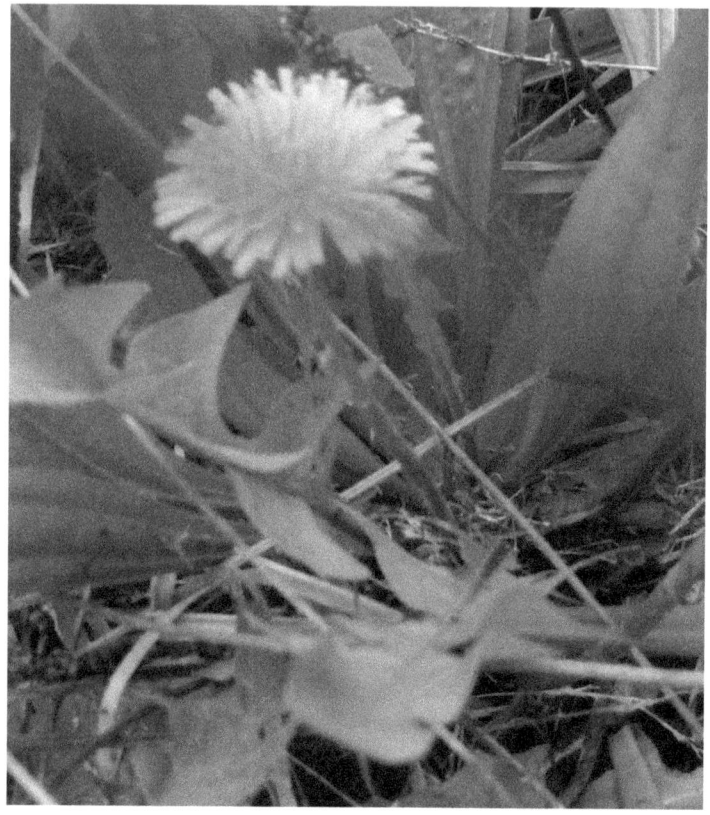

Echinacea ~ Echinacea, or Purple Coneflower, has long been used as an immune system booster. The most useful part of the plant is the root. You can make a decoction of it to drink or dry it and grind it into powder to make your own herbal capsules. You will want to make sure to use either Echinacea Purpura or

Echinacea Angustifolia, as these are the most common medicinal forms of Echinacea.

Elderberry ~ Elderberry syrup is commonly used for colds and flu. Elderberry is another good herb that is used as an immune system stimulant. Elderberries are rich in Vitamin C and have antiviral properties. They also seem to have expectorant and astringent properties that can help reduce congestion and get rid of phlegm.

Eucalyptus ~ Eucalyptus is most commonly used externally as an inhalation and vapor rub to treat and relieve mucus congestion. It can help with bronchitis, colds, flu and sinusitis. As an oil infusion it can be used for bruises, sprains, strains and various muscle pains.

Fennel ~ Fennel has restorative, cleansing, detoxifying and antiseptic properties. It helps maintain the elasticity of the skin because of an estrogen-like substance it contains. All parts of the plant can be used. Hippocrates even suggested using Fennel tea to increase the flow of breast milk in nursing mothers.

Feverfew ~ Feverfew is a good herb to treat headaches and even migraines. It is usually combined with other herbs in a medicinal tea because it has a bitter taste. It is often mistaken for Chamomile. It has proven to be the most effective if taken as you feel the headache or migraine coming on. It is anti-inflammatory due to its ability to hinder the production of prostaglandins which are hormone-like substances that cause pain and inflammation. Some studies have found that the anti-inflammatory effects of this Feverfew are even greater than those achieved by NSAIDs (Nonsteroidal anti-inflammatory drugs) such as Ibuprofen or Naproxen.

Garlic ~ Garlic can, and should, be eaten as food but it can also be used as a medicinal herb. Garlic has been shown to mildly lower blood pressure by dilating or expanding blood vessels. It also helps prevent blood clots, reducing the risk of heart attack and stroke, by decreasing the stickiness of platelets. When platelets are too sticky, they form clumps that can adhere to artery walls and contribute to clogged arteries. There are studies that also show it is helpful in reducing the pain and inflammation of arthritis, reducing the size of some cancerous tumors, preventing some forms of cancer.

Garlic is also antibiotic, antiviral, antifungal and antibacterial.

Ginkgo Biloba ~ The "Biloba" part of the name Ginkgo Biloba refers to the leaves that have two "lobes". It is a very distinct and easy to recognize plant. Ginkgo is antioxidant and a circulation stimulant. Today, it is most commonly used to increase memory. It improves blood circulation by opening the blood vessels and making the blood less sticky.

Ginkgo has been used to regulate blood flow to the brain but has also been shown to protect nerve cells that have been damaged by Alzheimer's disease. It has even been shown to help in cases of glaucoma, macular degeneration, leg pain and other circulatory problems.

Glycerine ~ Glycerine (sometimes seen as Glycerin) is derived from vegetable or animal sources (I use vegetable glycerine myself) and is a wonderful moisturizer and skin cleanser that softens and lubricates. Vegetable glycerine is hypoallergenic and easily soluble in water. Vegetable glycerine has a long shelf life and a sweet taste which is why it is ideal to make medicinal syrups for children.

Green Tea ~ Green Tea has become popular in recent years because of its antioxidant properties. It is also popular belief that Green Tea has anti-aging properties. It can be used as a face rinse to tighten the pores.

Honey ~ Honey has many wonderful properties. It is antibacterial, emollient, moisturizing, nourishing, soothing and cleansing. It also promotes healing. In ancient times it was thought to be "the food of the Gods" and what made them immortal. The Romans believed that using Honey on your skin made you more attractive especially when mixed with Olive Oil. Honey is one of the best known humectants and is high in Potassium, therefore making it difficult for bacteria to survive in it. Also, if you want to sweeten your medicinal teas you should use Honey instead of Sugar. Sugar has components in it that break down the medicinal properties in the teas and make them no longer work.

Honey, on the other hand, does not and is healthier for you than Sugar as well. Try to get organic raw Honey for the best results.

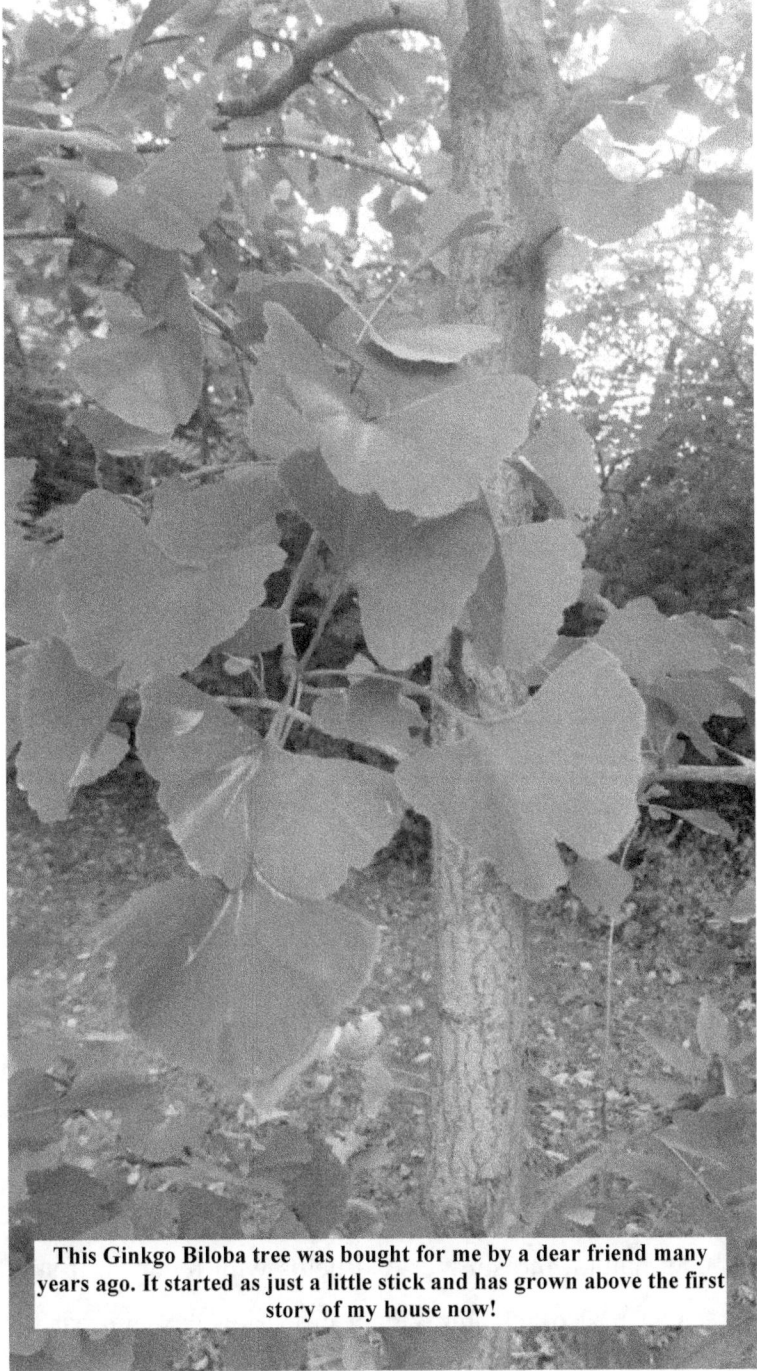

This Ginkgo Biloba tree was bought for me by a dear friend many years ago. It started as just a little stick and has grown above the first story of my house now!

Hops ~ Hops flowers are often used in a similar fashion to Valerian. They can be helpful for anxiety, insomnia, restlessness, tension, nervousness and irritability. Hops flowers are what gives beer its bitter flavor and are often used as a bitter tonic. They can lose their medicinal properties very quickly if exposed to light when stored.

Horehound ~ A good cough suppressant and expectorant is Horehound. It can be used as a syrup, a lozenge, a tea, etc to loosen phlegm from the chest. It contains a compound known as marrubiin which stimulates bronchial secretions and helps to break up congestion. It has been used for generations as a cure for children's cough, cold and croup. My grandmother used to tell me that when she was a little girl she loved eating Horehound candies. It may also be used to treat a mild upset stomach in children.

Jojoba Oil ~ Jojoba is very similar to the natural oil (known as sebum) that is secreted by your skin daily. Because of this, it is easily absorbed by the skin. Jojoba is a natural moisturizer and helps with renewal of skin cells. It also has antioxidant properties and is great for treating acne and problems such as eczema, psoriasis and dry skin.

Lavender ~ Lavender is one of my most favorite herbs. It is one of the few essential oils you can use neat (by itself, without diluting in a carrier oil) on the skin. It has so many wonderful properties as well; anti-inflammatory, antibacterial, antiseptic, balancing, relaxing, soothing. It helps both dry and oily skin by helping to normalize secretions from the sebaceous glands. It also stimulates growth of new cells. It can be used to repel insects as well as to calm yourself and reduce stress. Lavender can also help with sinus issues and headaches. If you are having trouble with either one take a couple drops of Lavender oil and put them on your temples and just under your eyes around the top of your cheek bones. This should help clear up the issue in no time.

Lemon ~ Lemon has antiseptic, rejuvenating, stimulating, astringent and mild bleaching properties. It also helps to restore the natural acid balance of the skin because it contains Citric Acid which is an AHA or alpha hydroxy acid and BHA or beta hydroxy acid.

Citric Acid also kills bacteria on the skin. Be careful though because citrus oils may irritate sensitive skins and cause photosensitivity (increased sensitivity to sunlight). Also, don't use on sore or irritated skin. The scent of Lemon is used in aromatherapy for its uplifting and refreshing effects.

Lemon Balm ~ Also known as Bee Balm or Melissa (its Latin name is Melissa Officinalis), Lemon Balm is part of the Mint family and is said to be antiviral. Studies have shown that putting a salve of Lemon Balm on herpes sores can make a huge difference in healing them.

Lemon Balm has also been used for digestive issues such as bloating, flatulence (gas), vomiting as well as menstrual cramps, headache, anxiety, restlessness, sleep disorders, ADHD, high blood pressure, sores and insect bites.

Due to its strong Lemon smell, Lemon Balm is excellent for adding to insect repellent recipes.

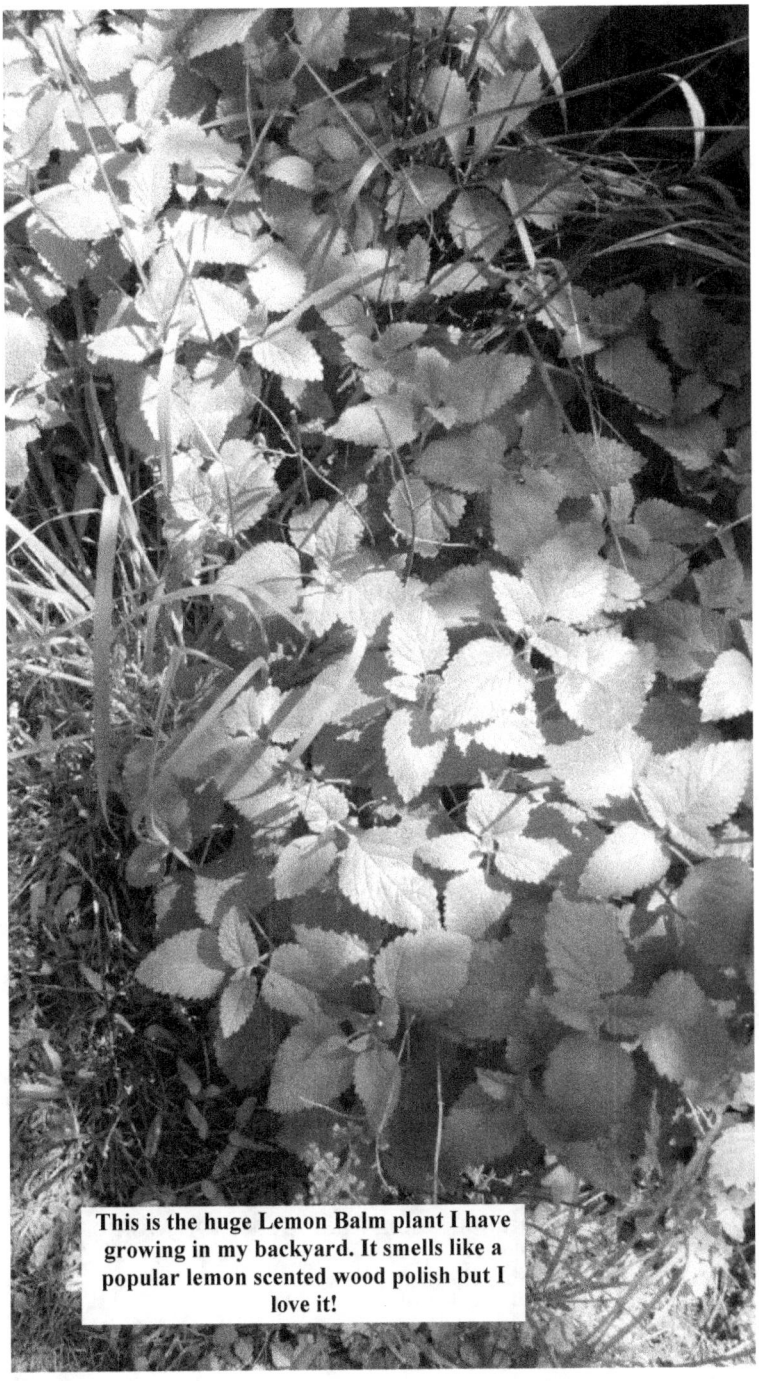

This is the huge Lemon Balm plant I have growing in my backyard. It smells like a popular lemon scented wood polish but I love it!

Lemon Verbena ~ Lemon Verbena, sometimes called Vervain, has been used for indigestion, gas, diarrhea, constipation, joint pain, insomnia, colds, fevers and varicose veins. It is most commonly used as a flavoring agent due to its extremely strong Lemony smell.

Lemongrass ~ Lemongrass is said to be antifungal, analgesic, astringent and can increase circulation.

Mint ~ Members of the Mint family tend to be naturally astringent as well as refreshing. They are good to use to boost your mood or wake you up. Some members of the Mint family are Spearmint, Peppermint, Wintergreen and Catnip.

Mullein ~ The Mullein plant is very good for problems related to breathing and congestion. You can drink Mullein tea to break up the mucus that clogs the lungs. You can also combine Mullein with garlic in an oil infusion to make a wonderful oil for ear infections. In ancient times Mullein leaves were used as diapering material for infants, menstrual pads for women and toilet tissue due to their softness.

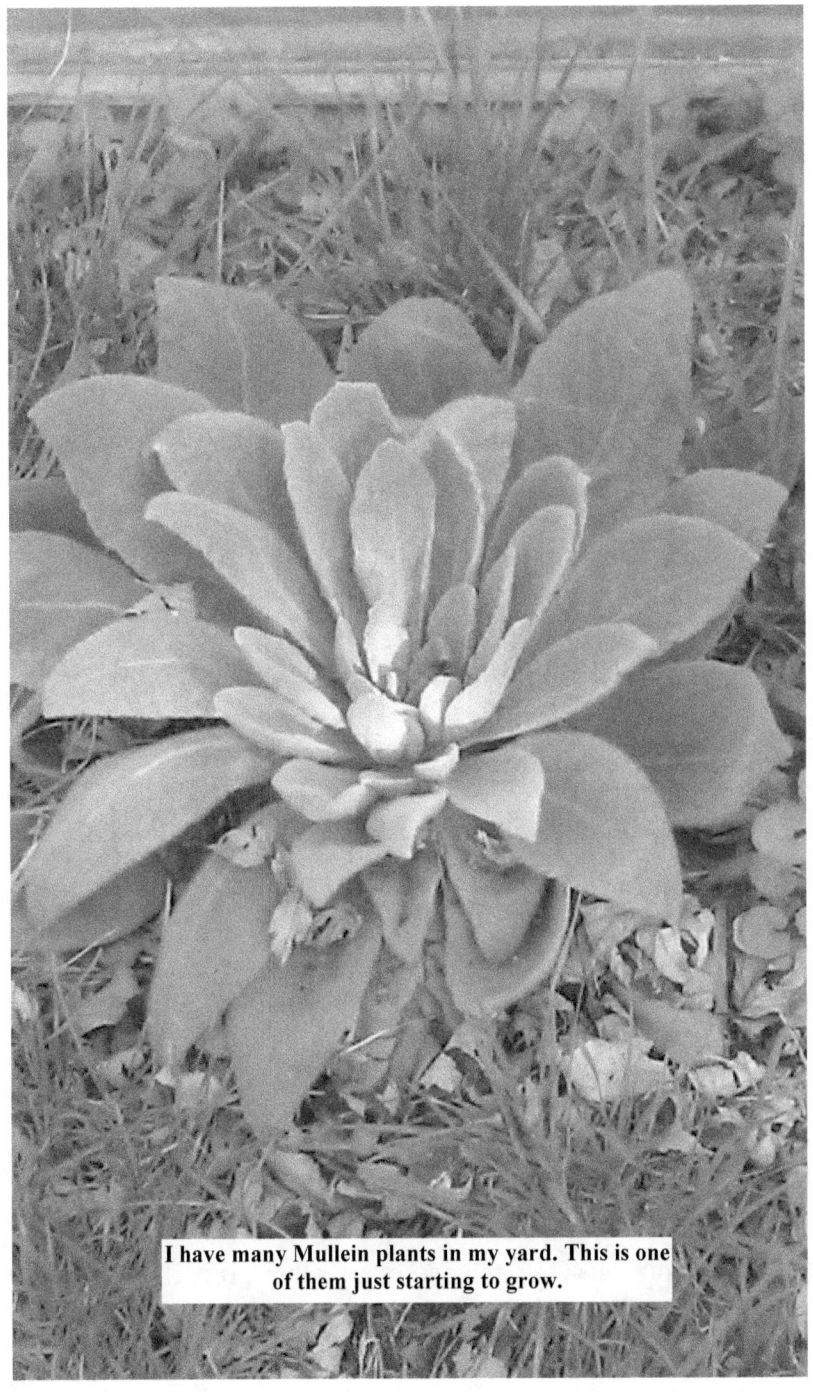

I have many Mullein plants in my yard. This is one of them just starting to grow.

Nettle ~ Nettle leaf, also known as Stinging Nettle, is best used fresh. It is full of nutrients and is often used to help with women's hormonal imbalances. You can make it into a tea or you can dry it and make your own herbal capsules. It is said to stimulate hair growth and is good for bronchial and asthmatic issues. I have heard of using the whole plant for arthritis pains by brushing the leaves over the afflicted area.

Olive Oil ~ Olive Oil is often used as an emollient and it attracts moisture to the skin. It has a long shelf life and blends well with other oils. I like to use Extra Virgin Olive Oil. You can often store Olive Oil, without refrigeration, for up to a year. It is especially good for dry skin and makes and excellent conditioner for nails and hair.

Onion ~ Onions are antibacterial and pull impurities from the skin. For example, if you are stung by a bee or bitten by an insect you can cut an onion in half and hold it on the wound for about 10 minutes. You'll want to do this as soon as possible to get as much of the toxins out as you can. Onions have many other properties as well. They can be used to aid digestion, help prevent hardening of the arteries, treat sore throats, bronchitis and asthma, among other things. They are a useful food and medicine to have around. Onions have even shown benefits in treating some forms of cancer.

Parsley ~ Parsley, like the members of the Mint family, is naturally astringent. It can also be soothing and healing for those who suffer with bad cases of acne, eczema and psoriasis. Ever wonder why restaurants put Parsley as a garnish on the plates? It's not just there to look pretty. Parsley freshens your breath after a meal. Parsley also makes a good rinse for all hair types.

Plantain ~ This common yard "weed" is actually very useful. It can be used in creams or salves to help heal minor scrapes and cuts. I have used it directly on the skin to help stop the bleeding of a wound. Plantain is abundant everywhere. It can be found all around urban areas. It is rich in Vitamin A, C, and K as well as Magnesium.

According to GreenMedInfo.com "Studies have shown that plantain has anti-inflammatory effects, and it is also rich in tannins (which helps draw tissues together to stop bleeding) and allantoin (a compound that promotes healing of injured skin cells). Further studies have indicated that plantain may also reduce blood pressure, and that the seeds of the plant may reduce blood cholesterol levels. Plantain seeds were also widely used as a natural laxative, given their high source of fiber. Teas made from the plant, were used to treat diarrhea, dysentery, intestinal worms, and bleeding mucous membranes. The roots were also recommended for relieving toothaches and headaches as well as healing poor gums."

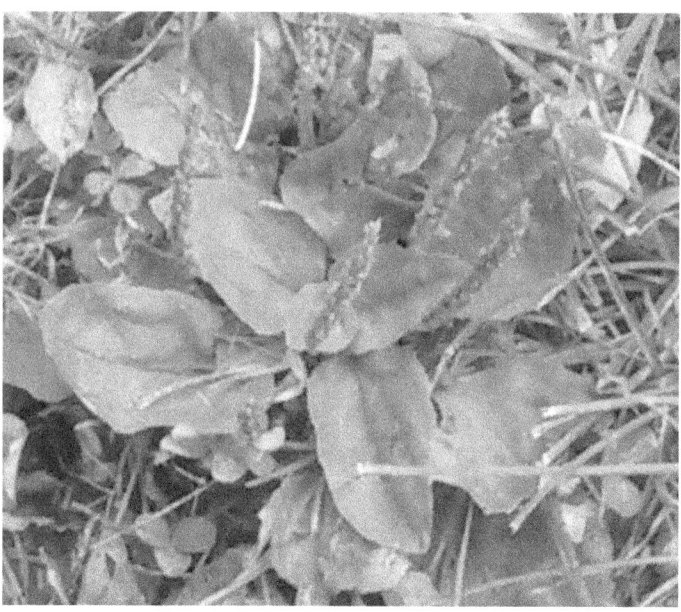

Peppermint ~ Peppermint is invigorating, cooling, anti-inflammatory, analgesic and mildly antiseptic. It's good for helping to get rid of aches and pains as well as controlling bacteria on the skin.

Raspberry ~ Raspberry leaf tea has been used to help many women's issues. It is said to help with hormone imbalances, menstrual cramps as well as childbirth. You can find it often combined with Nettle.

Rose ~ Roses have long been associated with love and beauty. The essence of Roses has been used for centuries for such things as relieving Depression and grief, attracting love and passion, as an aphrodisiac as well as symbolizing beauty. Some say that Rose oil is one of the first essential oils documented for use. You can use them to make Rose water which can be a wonderful toner to the skin, especially when combined with glycerine. If you decide that you would like to try to make your own Rose water make sure to use organically grown Roses so that you won't be adding pesticides and other harsh chemicals to your skin.

Rosemary ~ Rosemary has astringent, antiseptic, anti-inflammatory, nervine, carminative, diuretic, antidepressant, circulatory stimulant, antispasmodic, detoxifying and stimulating properties. It helps to rid the skin of impurities by opening the pores and helps to prevent wrinkles. It is very helpful for oily skin and is a strong antioxidant. Rosemary is known to improve circulation as well as promoting hair growth, conditioning hair and preventing dandruff. It is a good herb to use in sore or sprained muscle rubs.

Dried Rosemary leaves from my spice cabinet.

Sage ~ Sage has been used to darken and tone hair as well as being a hair growth stimulant. It also has antibacterial properties. Sage has been used for its carminative (anti-gas) properties as well as to relieve stomach pain, diarrhea, bloating, heartburn, Depression and memory loss. It can be used to slow milk production in mothers and to reduce hot flashes caused by menopause.

Tea Tree – Tea Tree Oil is also known as Melaleuca oil and is native to Australia. It is my second favorite oil, next to Lavender. It is antiseptic, antifungal, antibacterial and antiviral. It is easily absorbed by the skin and, along with Lavender, can be used neat (by itself, without diluting in a carrier oil). I use a few drops of it in shampoo to help with dandruff. Tea Tree has been used as an antiseptic, fungicide and germicide.

Thyme ~ Thyme is antifungal, antiseptic, anti-inflammatory, anti-parasitic, expectorant, an immune booster and also is a lung cleanser. Because of its expectorant and lung cleansing properties it is often used for whooping cough, bronchitis, asthma and other ailments related to breathing and/or congestion. It used to be given, in tea form, to women who had just given birth in order to expel the placenta. It can also be made into a paste by mashing up the fresh leaves, or dried leaves combined with water or other liquid, and applied as a poultice.

Turmeric ~ This is a spice that should be easy to find in your local grocery store. It is often used to prevent wrinkles due to its anti-allergic, antiseptic, antioxidant and nerve and blood vessel stimulating properties.

Valerian ~ The root of the Valerian plant is the most commonly used. It is touted as a nervine and a sedative. It can be used for someone who suffers from anxiety issues or to help you get to sleep at night. It helps to reduce stress, nervous tension, Depression, irritability, hysteria, panic, anxiety, fear, stomach cramping, indigestion due to nervousness, delusions, exhaustion, and, of course, nervous sleeplessness. It is even said to help in cases of sciatica, multiple sclerosis, epilepsy, shingles, and peripheral neuropathy, including numbness, tingling, muscle weakness, and pain in the extremities. It has been said that it can even help with behavioral problems in both adults and children, and is used to treat attention deficit disorders, hyperactivity and anxiety headaches. I have used it myself to help treat a child with Attention Deficit Hyperactivity Disorder (ADHD).

Witch Hazel ~ Many of you may be familiar with Witch Hazel already but did you know it has toning, astringent, antiseptic and anti-inflammatory properties? It is soothing to irritated skin and doesn't dry it out. It also helps to prevent wrinkles by toning and refreshing the skin. It is much better to use on oily skin than alcohol which dries the skin out and can cause it to produce even more oil.

Yarrow ~ Yarrow is astringent and anti-inflammatory. It is used often with acne prone skin. It can also be used as a sitz bath for those suffering from hemorrhoids. It can be used on wounds to help stop bleeding. I like to make a salve with it, combined with Plantain, to help with minor cuts, scrapes and bruises.

How to make Salves by Starr Morgayne

Products You Can Purchase

You can purchase these products and more by checking out https://www.etsy.com/shop/NaturalSelectionWB

None of these items have been evaluated by the FDA and are not intended to diagnose, cure, or treat any ailment or illness. We also take requests for custom blends.

Sole Soothing Foot Lotion $10 + S&H
8 oz bottle with pump top (shape and color may vary)

This lotion feels great and works even better. Being a Diabetic I was looking for something that would soften the rough skin on my heels. After searching and searching I finally decided to take matters into my own hands. I created this lotion and have never looked back. It contains Aloe Vera, Cocoa Butter and Calendula Petals to soften and heal the skin. It also contains Comfrey leaves for their skin rejuvenating properties. I've also added Tea Tree and Lavender Oils for their antifungal, antiseptic and antibiotic attributes along with Peppermint Oil for its cooling and circulatory benefits.
Ingredients: Aloe Vera Juice, Cocoa Butter, Vegetable glycerine, Olive Oil, Emulsifying Wax, Calendula Petals, Comfrey Leaves, Lavender Buds, Lavender Essential Oil, Tea Tree Essential Oil, Peppermint Essential Oil

ACE Face and Eye Cream $5 + S&H
2 oz walled jar with lid (color may vary)

This natural skin cream is perfect for revitalizing maturing skin or maintaining younger looking skin. It contains vitamins A, C, and E mixed in Coconut Oil to enhance the elasticity in your skin. It repairs skin tissue and damage. It softens skin, moisturizes, and reduces the appearance of scarring, wrinkles, and stretch marks. I have had some great reviews on its benefits for those with Rosacea also!

Ingredients: Organic extra virgin Coconut Oil, glycerine, water, Vitamin E, Vitamin C, Vitamin A

All Natural Antibiotic First Aid Ointment $3 + S&H
¼ oz container with lid

This is a first aid ointment or salve that can be used for cuts, scrapes, bruises, abrasions, etc. It was made using all natural ingredients.

The herbs used in this product are used for these purposes:
• Tea Tree Oil: antibiotic, anti-fungal, antiviral, antibacterial
• Lavender: analgesic (pain relief), antibiotic, anti-fungal, antiviral, antibacterial
• Lemon: antibiotic, antifungal, antiviral, antibacterial
Ingredients: Extra Virgin Olive Oil, Beeswax, Vitamin E, Lavender Essential Oil, Tea Tree Essential Oil, Lemon Essential Oil, Calendula Petals, Comfrey Leaf

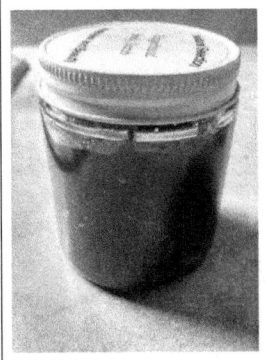

Gingerbread Body Scrub $5 + S&H
4 oz glass jar with lid

This is an all natural body scrub that smells heavenly. Perfect for a gift for yourself or someone you love. Extra Virgin Olive Oil is a great moisturizer for the skin. Sugar is an excellent exfoliant and the spices used in this scrub can help with circulation. As with all products, some settling may occur. Just stir and use.

Ingredients: Brown Sugar, Cinnamon, Nutmeg, Ginger, Cloves, essential oils, Extra Virgin Olive Oil, Sugar

Pumpkin Pie Body Scrub $5 + S&H
4 oz walled jar with lid

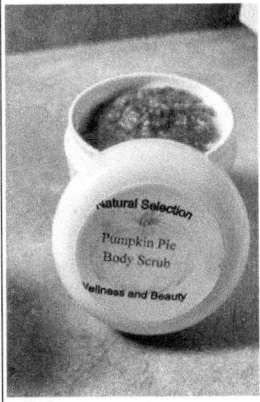

This is an all natural body scrub that smells heavenly. Perfect for a gift for yourself or someone you love. Coconut Oil and Honey are great moisturizers for the skin. Sugar is an excellent exfoliant and the spices used in this scrub can help with circulation. As with all products, some settling may occur. Just stir and use. Due to the fact that this body scrub contains Coconut Oil it will solidify at lower temperatures.

Ingredients: Coconut Oil, brown Sugar, Honey, pumpkin pie spices, Cinnamon, Nutmeg, Ginger

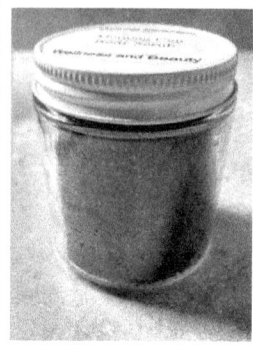

Morning Cup Body Scrub $5 + S&H
4 oz glass jar with lid

This is a wonderful body scrub that will invigorate you! The coffee and the Peppermint in this scrub will wake you right up. The caffeine in the coffee grounds has also been shown to reduce the appearance and formation of cellulite so there's an added bonus! Great for every morning, especially those mornings when you just can't seem to rise and shine.

Ingredients: Coffee beans, Olive Oil, Peppermint Essential Oil, Salt

Cleansing Grains Face Scrub $4 + S&H
2 oz glass jar with lid

This facial scrub is gentle on sensitive facial skin but great for exfoliating. Combine a little with water or whole milk and scrub gently to reduce redness, oil, puffiness and signs of aging.

Ingredients: Oats, Almonds, Rose petals, Lavender, Kaolin clay

Soothing Burn Spray $8 + S&H
4 oz spray bottle

This is an excellent spray for any type of burn. If stored in the refrigerator it adds a refreshing coolness to the spray. Excellent for spraying on sunburns or other minor burns or wounds.

Bottle color may vary.

Ingredients: Aloe Vera Juice, Lavender Essential Oil, Vitamin E

Lavender Milk Bath $10 + S&H
Wooden corked bottle with spoon

Milk is a soothing, moisturizing, yet non-greasy bath additive that gently soothes and cleanses your child's skin. A warm Lavender aromatherapy bath does wonders for a fussy baby or toddler (or even Mommy). Comes in a gorgeous glass jar with a wooden lid and wooden spoon attached on the side.

To use: Use the little wooden spoon to sprinkle a small amount in a warm bath

Ingredients: Lavender, milk, cornstarch

How to make Salves by Starr Morgayne

Companies

Natural Selection Wellness and Beauty
P.O. Box 11496
Fort Wayne, Indiana 46858-1496
USA
https://www.etsy.com/people/naturalselectionwb
NaturalSelectionWB@gmail.com

THAYERS Natural Remedies
P.O. Box 56
Westport, Connecticut 06881-0056
USA
http://www.thayers.com

Mountain Rose Herbs
P.O. Box 50220
Eugene, OR 97405
USA
http://www.mountainroseherbs.com

Frontier Natural Foods Co-op
P.O. Box 299
3021 78th St.
Norway, IA 52318
USA
http://www.frontiercoop.com/

Index

infusion, 12, 17, 18, 20,
21, 44, 47, 49, 54
infusions, 6, 7, 10, 14,
23, 47, 51, 52, 114
inhalation, 65
insect bites, 72
insect repellent, 72
insomnia, 70, 74
intestinal, 78
invigorating, 79
irritability, 70, 82
irritated skin, 72
Jojoba Oil, 7, 8, 9, 70
Kaolin clay, 88
lard, 25, 26
Lavender, 31, 32, 33,
35, 48, 71, 81, 85, 86,
88, 89
laxative, 59, 78
leaves, 11, 36, 37, 59,
63, 67, 74, 76, 80, 82,
85
Lemon, 35, 36, 71, 72,
74, 86

Lemon Balm, 36, 72
Lemon Verbena, 74
Lemongrass, 74
lip balm, 31, 36, 37
liver, 59, 64
lotion, 17, 45, 85
lotions, 3, 9, 24, 52, 55,
63
lozenge, 70
lung, 81
lungs, 74
lymph nodes, 57
maceration, 47
macular degeneration,
67
Magnesium, 77
Marigold, 59
marinade, 23
massage, 7, 9, 24, 55,
57
mature skin, 9, 57
medicinal, 51, 65, 66,
67, 68, 70
medicine, 3, 40, 63, 77

Suggested Reading

Here are several books that I would recommend for doing some research on your own. This is by no means an extensive list.

Buhner, Stephen Harrod, *Herbal Antibiotics; Natural Alternatives for Treating Drug-Resistant Bacteria*, Storey Books, 1999

Foster, Steven, *101 Medicinal Herbs; An Illustrated Guide*, Interweave Press, 1998

Gladstar, Rosemary, *Herbal Healing for Women; Simple Home Remedies for Women of All Ages*, Simon & Schuster, 1993

Keville, Kathi, *Herbs for Health and Healing*, Rodale Press, Inc., 1996

Kowalchik, Claire and Hylton, William H. (editors), *Rodale's Illustrated Encyclopedia of Herbs*, Rodale Press, 1987

Mars, Brigitte, Herbalist AHG, *Dandelion Medicine; Remedies and Recipes to Detoxify, Nourish, Stimulate*, Storey Books, 1999

Morgayne, Starr, *Bewitching Beauty; Bringing out your inner Goddess, naturally*, Dark Moon Press, 2010

Morgayne, Starr, *How To Make Infusions and Decoctions*, Dark Moon Press, 2014

Murray, Michael N.D. and Pizzorno, Joseph N.D., *Encyclopedia of Natural Medicine*, Revised 2nd Edition, Prima Publishing, 1998

Rose, Jeanne, *Herbs & Aromatherapy for the Reproductive System*, Frog Ltd., 1994

Royal, Penny C., *Herbally Yours*, Third Edition, Sound Nutrition, 1982

Smyth, Angela, *The Complete Home Healer; Your Guide to Every Treatment Available for over 300 of the Most Common Health Problems*, HarperCollins Publishers, 1994

Telesco, Patricia, *The Herbal Arts; A Handbook of Gardening, Recipes, Healing, Crafts, and Spirituality,* Carol Publishing Group, 1998

Trattler, Dr. Ross, N.D., D.O., *Better Health through Natural Healing; How To Get Well Without Drugs or Surgery,* Second Edition, Hinkler Books Pty Ltd, 2001

Walker, Dr. Lynne Paige and Brown, Ellen Hodgson J.D., *Nature's Pharmacy; Break the Drug Cycle with Safe Natural Treatments for 200 Everyday Ailments,* Reward Books, 1998

Weed, Susun S, *Wise Woman Herbal for the Childbearing Year,* Ash Tree Publishing, 1986

White, Linda B., M.D. and Mavor, Sunny A.H.G, *Kids, Herbs, Health,* Interweave Press, 1998

About the Author

Starr Morgayne is in her thirties and has been studying herbs and alternative healing methods for more than 15 years. She is a Certified Herbalist and is working to obtain a degree in Naturopathy.

She lives in Indiana with her four cats, three dogs, two ferrets, lots of fish and her loving family.

In her spare time she enjoys writing, reading, photography, crafting and gardening.

Dark Moon Press
P.O. Box 11496
Fort Wayne, Indiana 46858-1496
DarkMoon@darkmoonpress.com
www.darkmoonpress.com

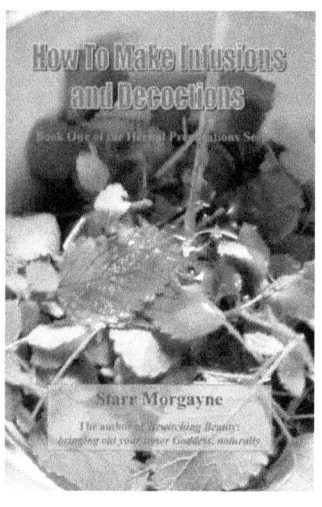

How to make Infusions and Decoctions; Book One of the Herbal Preparations Series
Starr Morgayne

Starr Morgayne returns with her newest release as she instructs the reader on her secrets of making herbal infusions and other remedies from her kitchen to yours. In this book she describes how to make bath teas, steam facials, instructs you in how to make herbal syrups and much more. This herbalist has taken photos from her own herb garden to show the plants in bloom and clearly illustrate how she creates simple to make, yet effective, treatments such as clove toothache oil, mullein and garlic ear oil and a wide variety of teas.
ISBN-13: 978-1493503650
113 pages
$9.99 USD

Walking the Path of the Ancient Ways; a collection of magic by various pagan authors
Corvis Nocturnum

Pagan authors from various backgrounds share their story on being pagan in the modern world. Insightful and thought provoking. With writings by Starr Morgayne, Corvis Nocturnum, Andrieh Vitimus and many more known and new voices.
ISBN-13: 978-1470034641
200 pages
9.99 USD

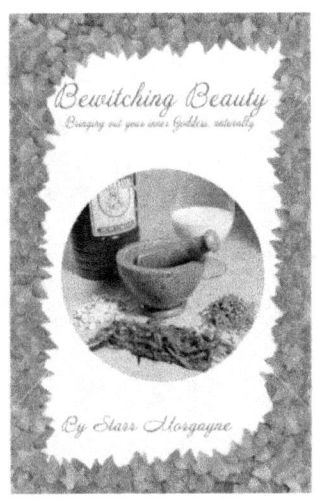

Bewitching Beauty: Bringing out your inner Goddess, naturally
Starr Morgayne

Women of all ages are concerned about their skin, their bodies and growing older. In this book the author offers simple yet effective, personally tested recipes based on readily available ingredients, and her own unique perspective to help get you in touch with Mother Nature and yourself. Regardless of what stage of life you are in this book can be a positive addition to your journey.
ISBN-13: 978-1451585872
200 pages
$16.95 USD

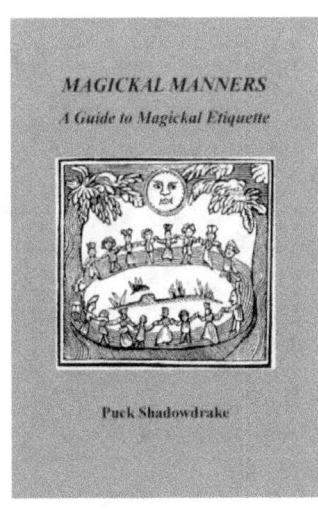

MAGICKAL MANNERS: A Guide to Magickal Etiquette
Puck Shadowdrake

"An extensive overview of the practices and etiquette of the entire Neo Pagan community. An excellent resource for chaplains as well as for students seeking a spiritual path." Kerr Cuhulain, author of *Pagan Religions: A Handbook for Diversity Training*
ISBN-13: 978-1481910958
600 pages
$39.99 USD

JOURNEYS FROM THE MEADOW: A Book of Guided
Mediations
Puck Shadowdrake

Puck Shadowdrake, the author of *MAGICKAL MANNERS: A
Guide to Magickal Etiquette* brings you his collection of
meditations to guide the modern witch through their various
journeys through the path for relaxation, healing the body and
contacting your deities, spirit guides and much more.
Pages: TBA
Price: $19.99 USD
Spring 2015